I0414123

Keto Chips:
35 Best Recipes of Low Carb Chips to Satisfy Your Crunchy-Savory Craving

Disclamer: All photos used in this book, including the cover photo were made available under a Attribution-ShareAlike 2.0 Generic (CC BY-SA 2.0)

and sourced from Flickr

Copyright 2016 by publisher - All rights reserved.

This document is geared towards providing exact and reliable information in regards to the topic and issue covered. The publication is sold with the idea that the publisher is not required to render accounting, officially permitted, or otherwise, qualified services. If advice is necessary, legal or professional, a practiced individual in the profession should be ordered.

- From a Declaration of Principles which was accepted and approved equally by a Committee of the American Bar Association and a Committee of Publishers and Associations.

In no way is it legal to reproduce, duplicate, or transmit any part of this document in either electronic means or in printed format. Recording of this publication is strictly prohibited and any storage of this document is not allowed unless with written permission from the publisher. All rights reserved.

The information provided herein is stated to be truthful and consistent, in that any liability, in terms of inattention or otherwise, by any usage or abuse of any policies, processes, or directions contained within is the solitary and utter responsibility of the recipient reader. Under no circumstances will any legal responsibility or blame be held against the publisher for any reparation, damages, or monetary loss due to the information herein, either directly or indirectly.

Respective authors own all copyrights not held by the publisher.

The information herein is offered for informational purposes solely, and is universal as so. The presentation of the information is without contract or any type of guarantee assurance.

The trademarks that are used are without any consent, and the publication of the trademark is without permission or backing by the trademark owner. All trademarks and brands within this book are for clarifying purposes only and are the owned by the owners themselves, not affiliated with this document.

Table of conten

Introduction.

The Keto diet involves going long spells on extremely low (no higher than 30g per day) to almost zero-g per day of carbs and increasing your fats to a high level (to the point where they may make up as much as 65% of your daily macronutrients intake.) The idea is to get your body into a state of ketosis. In this state of ketosis, the body is supposed to be more inclined to use fat for energy- and research says it does just this. Depleting your carbohydrate/glycogen liver stores and then moving onto fat for fuel means you should end up being shredded.

Benefits of Keto Diet

Lower blood sugar and insulin levels – helping to prevent and manage diabetes

When carbs are consumed, they are broken down into glucose, increasing the blood sugar levels. The body responds by releasing insulin (to lower blood sugar levels). Unfortunately, if you overload your body continuously with sugar (as a result of insulin), the cells in your body becomes resistant to the insulin. Your body's natural process to reduce your blood sugar is reduced, hence your blood sugar remains unnaturally high. This is type II diabetes.

So what's the simple solution to bringing your blood sugar down? Do not eat carbs (which produce the sugar). One study suggested diabetics on a low carb diet can reduce their insulin dosage by 50% (1).

Lower blood sugar also results in feeling better. Remember when you have a big lunch then feel sleepy for the rest of the afternoon? That was because of a spike in your blood sugar.

Suppressing your appetite

On a Ketogenic diet you feel fuller, which means you crave food (including junk food), far less. This then becomes a simple equation, if you feel like eating less, you eat less. Eating less ultimately leads to weight loss.

Greater fat loss – particularly the stubborn belly fat

Potentially one of the best benefits of the ketogenic diet is increased fat loss around the stomach area. Shedding this visceral fat around the mid region was always something I struggled with and I began to see a significant reduction in fat on a ketogenic diet. One study which compared a low fat and a low carb diet was surprised at this finding:

Both between and within group comparisons revealed a distinct advantage of a VLCK (low carb) over a LF (low fat) diet for weight loss, total fat loss, and trunk fat loss for men' (2)

They also highlighted the trunk loss in women, but it was not as significant as within men (women tend to store fat more proportionally around the body).

The loss of visceral (internal) fat helps to reduce the chances of diabetes and general health problems in the future.

Lower levels of triglycerides

Triglycerides are fat in your blood. You may think this is a bad thing, but they are needed to provide energy around the body. If you have too many of them, however, your body saves them for a rainy day somewhere around your body as fat. High levels also lead to a higher chance of diabetes and heart disease.

One of the biggest contributing factors to high levels is simple sugars. Cutting out these sugars reduces your triglyceride levels.

Increase in good cholesterol and a decrease in bad cholesterol

At one point, all cholesterol was considered bad, however within recent years it has been proven that there is good and bad cholesterol.

LDL (low density lipoprotein) is the bad stuff, while HDL (high density lipoprotein) is the good stuff.

HDL carries cholesterol from the rest of the body for processing, where it is used or 'thrown away'. LDL can clot and form fatty deposits, blocking arteries (contributing to heart conditions and increased blood pressure).

Studies have shown one of the best ways to increase HDL levels and reduce LDL levels is a high fat diet.

Increased mental focus

Low carb diets were one of the earliest forms of treatment for epilepsy (until more effective drugs were developed). The diet is also now being explored as a way to treat and stave off Alzheimer's and Parkinson's disease.

Fatty acids (particularly omega 3 and 6) are considered beneficial for cognitive functioning and help you keep more focused and alert.

RECIPES

1. Baked Beetroot Chips

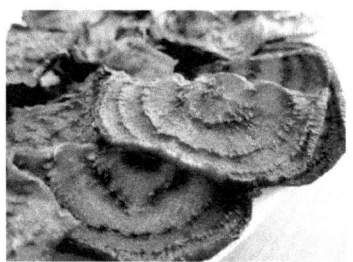

These healthy beetroot chips make a colorful addition to the selection of snacks you offer your family and friends.

Ingredients for 2 servings

- 2 Large Beetroots

- 2 tbsp. Virgin Olive Oil

- 1/2 tsp. Sea Salt

Preparation – 20 to 25 minutes

1. Preheat the oven to 360 F (180 C).

2. Wash the beetroots thoroughly and then peel them.

3. Using the lowest (thinnest) setting on your mandolin slice the beetroots into rounds.

4. Drizzle 1 tbsp. of virgin olive oil on a baking tray.

5. Place the beetroot rounds on the baking tray and drizzle the remaining 1 tbsp. of virgin olive oil on top and lightly season with the sea salt.

6. When the oven is at temperature place the baking tray in the oven and bake for 15 to 20 minutes. Turn the chips over after 8 to 10 minutes.

7. When the edges of the beetroot appear to be crispy they are ready to be removed from the oven.

8. Let the beetroot chips cool for a couple of minutes and then serve.

2. Classic Kale Chips

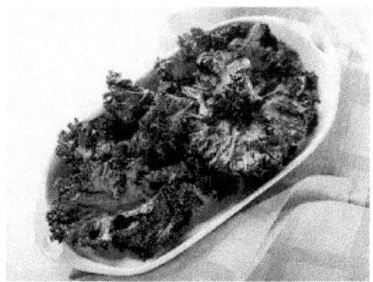

These kale chips are rich in iron, vitamin K, and antioxidants. Delicious, crispy and healthy!

Ingredients for 2-3 servings

- 1 Large Head of Green Kale

- 2 tbsp. Virgin Olive Oil

- 1/2 tsp. Sea Salt

Preparation – 25 to 30 minutes

1. Preheat the oven to 300 F (150 C).

2. Wash the Kale leaves with cold fresh water and then pat them dry.

3. Remove the stems from the Kale leaves and discard them.

4. Tear the Kale leaves into pieces.

5. In a large bowl drizzle 1 tbsp. of virgin olive oil over the torn up kale leaves and toss thoroughly.

6. Drizzle 1 tbsp. of virgin olive oil onto a baking tray.

7. Place the kale leaves evenly over the baking tray and put into the now hot oven and bake for 20 to 25 minutes. Turn the chips over after 10 to 15 minutes.

8. Remove the baking tray from the oven and set aside to cool for approximately 5 minutes.

9. With a plastic spatula remove the now cool kale chips from the baking tray and serve. Note that if you try to remove the kale leaves whilst they are still hot they will crumble. If this happens just let them cool a little longer.

3. Tasty Taro Chips

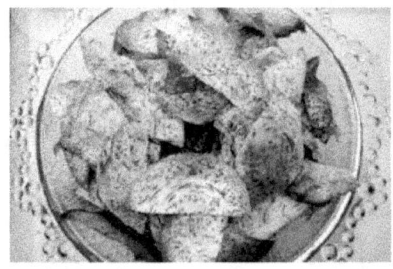

The natural sugars in this south Asian vegetable give a sweet nutty flavor to the chips.

Ingredients for 3-4 servings

- 1/2 lb. (225 grams) of Taro.

- 1 tbsp. Virgin Olive Oil

- 1 tsp. Sea Salt

Preparation – 25 to 30 minutes

1. Preheat the oven to 400 F (205 C).

2. Wash the Taro and then peel them.

3. Using the lowest (thinnest) setting on your mandoline slice the taro lengthwise.

4. Drizzle the virgin olive oil on a baking tray.

5. Place the taro slices on the baking tray and lightly season with the sea salt.

6. When the oven is at temperature place the baking tray in the oven and bake for 15 to 20 minutes. Turn the chips over after 8 to 10 minutes.

7. When the edges of the taro appear to be crispy they are ready to be removed from the oven.

8. Let the taro chips cool for a couple of minutes and then serve.

4. Baked Zucchini & Parmesan Chips

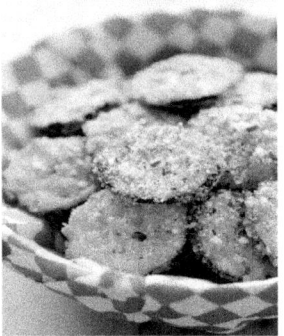

The combination of zucchini and Parmesan cheese leave a delightful tang in the mouth.

Ingredients for 4 servings

- 2 Zucchini (1 lb. or 454 grams approximately)

- 1/4 cup of Freshly grated Parmesan Cheese

- 1/4 cup Plain dry bread crumbs

- 1 tbsp. Virgin Olive Oil

- 1/2 tsp. Sea Salt

- 1/2 tsp. Ground black pepper

Preparation – 40 to 50 minutes

1. Preheat the oven to 450 F (230 C).

2. Wash the Zucchini.

3. Using your mandoline slice the zucchini into rounds approximately 1/4 inch (0.6 cm) thick.

4. Put the zucchini rounds into a large bowl along with the 1 tbsp. of virgin olive oil and toss thoroughly.

5. In a small bowl or a cup mix together the bread crumbs with the Parmesan cheese, salt and pepper.

6. Drizzle some virgin olive oil on a baking tray.

7. Dip each of the zucchini rounds into the Parmesan mixture making sure that the mixture sticks to both sides of the round.

8. Place each round onto the baking tray and put into the oven when at temperature.

9. Bake for 25 minutes until the zucchini rounds are crispy and brown. Turn the chips over after 12 to 15 minutes.

10. Remove the baking tray from the oven and remove the Zucchini chips with a plastic spatula.

11. Serve and enjoy!

5. Broccoli Chips

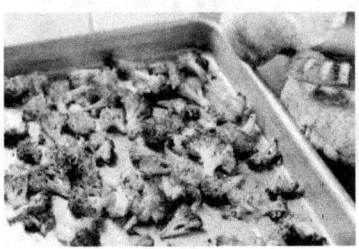

Required Ingredients:

1. Four broccoli stumps

2. Cooking spray

3. Salt to suit your taste

4. Black pepper to suit your taste

Method:

1. Keep an oven preheated at about 175 degrees Celsius.

2. Now cut the broccoli in the shape of circles or coins, as thin as possible.

3. You can use a slicer or slice them with a knife very carefully.

4. Now coat the thinly sliced broccoli with the cooking spray.

5. Place the chips on a baking sheet in a single layer.

6. Sprinkle a little salt and black pepper powder over the chips.

7. Bake the chips for about ten minutes, or until they are crisp enough.

8. Serve them hot or you can store them in a plastic bag.

6. *Zucchini Chips*

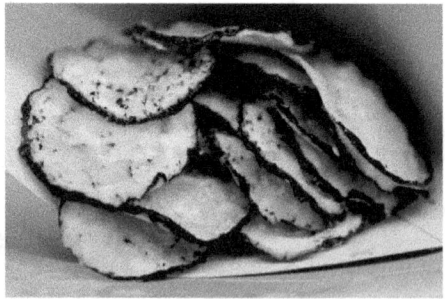

Required Ingredients:

1. Two cups zucchini, cut into extremely thin circles or coins

2. Half tablespoon canola oil, or olive oil, or any other edible oil

3. One-fourth cup finely very thinly grated cheese

4. Cooking spray

5. Salt and pepper to suit your taste

Method

1. Keep an oven preheated at about 180 degree Celsius.

2. Put the thinly sliced zucchini chips in a bowl and add the oil.

3. Coat the chips with the oil and drain off the excess oil if there is any left in the bowl.

4. Now pour the cheese over the chips and toss them thoroughly so that the chips are coated with the cheese.

5. Now spread the chips on the baking sheet and spray cooking spray over them. The chips should be placed in a single layer.

6. Now place the baking sheet with the chips in the preheated oven.

7. Bake them for fifteen minutes.

8. Flip the chips or coins to change their side.

9. Bake them again for about ten minutes, until they are crisp enough.

10. Do not overcook the chips. If they are overcooked they will become soggy.

7.Garlic Chips

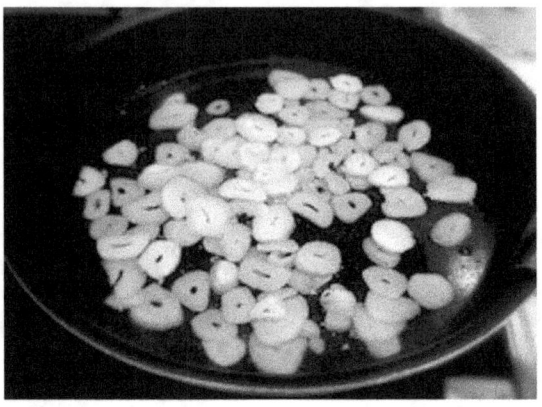

Required Ingredients

1. Peeled cloves of four garlic bulbs

2. Three tablespoons olive oil

3. One teaspoon black salt, or the normal salt

Method

1. Slice the garlic cloves in very thin circles or rounds, as thin as possible Heat the olive oil in a frying pan.

2. Add the garlic slices and spread them all over the surface of the pan in a single layer. Do not crush them.

3. Sauté the garlic slices for about ten minutes, until they are brown and crispy.

4. Now remove the chips from the frying pan and spread them over paper towels to drain off the excess oil.

5. Sprinkle the salt over the fried garlic slices and serve them with other snacks and drinks.

8. **Potato chips**

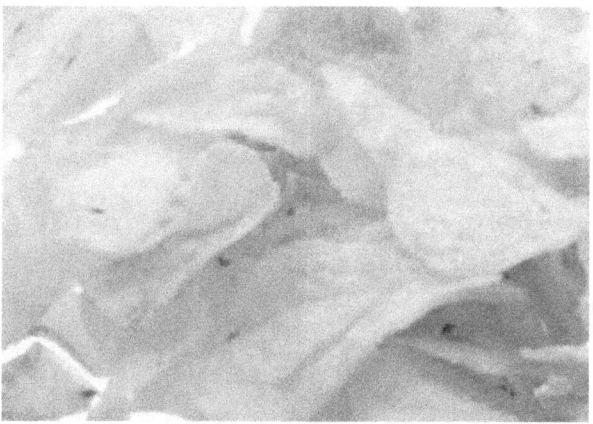

Please do not confuse potato chips with sweet potato chips when you have already learned about in the previous pages.

The potato chips are the most widely eaten chips all over the world. They are found in different flavors and tastes. They are cheap and they are found in different packets of different weights.

Potato chips are liked by both young and old because they are light and easy to digest. Follow the instructions and prepare potato chips in your own kitchen.

Required Ingredients

1. One kilo potatoes

2. Oil for frying

3. Salt to suit your taste

4. Hot water

5. Cold water

6. Half a teaspoon of dry mango powder

7. Half a teaspoon of allspices

Method

1. Peel the potatoes and put them in cold water for about half an hour. See that you have not taken sweet potatoes. You should have normal potatoes.

2. Now cut them into chips with a slicer or a sharp knife. If you are using a knife, slice the chips as thin as possible.

3. Put the sliced potatoes back into the cold water.

4. Now rub the chips with your hands inside the water to remove extra starch. Keep rubbing them inside the water for about five minutes.

5. Put the chips in another bowl filled with cold water. Add a little salt and leave them in the water for about ten minutes.

6. Now boil some water in a deep pan and when the water is hot put the potato slices into the water and let them simmer for about ten minutes over medium heat. Increase the heat and bring the water to a boil.

7. Remove the chips from the hot water and put them back into cold water. We do this to make chips crispy, and secondly they will not absorb much oil while frying.

8. Now heat the oil, about two to three inches, in a deep frying pan.

9. Remove the potato slices from the water and wipe them with a cotton cloth.

10. When the oil is hot, start leaving the potato slices into the oil in small batches. Deep fry them.

11. Mix some salt in a bowl of water and sprinkle this salted water over the chips that are still being fried. By doing this, the chips will become crispy.

12. Now remove the chips from the oil and place them on paper towels.

13. When the chips are cool enough, put them in a serving tray and sprinkle salt, a little mango powder and all-purpose spice according to your taste.

14. Serve them hot with tea or coffee. You can store these chips in an air-tight container after mixing the spices.

9. Taro Chips (Rabbi Chips)

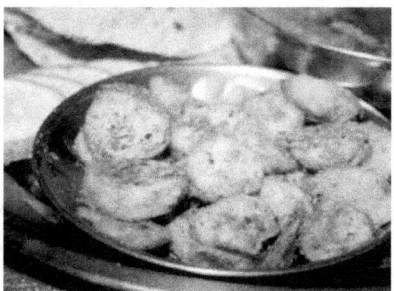

Required Ingredients

1. Half a kilo taro root (Rabbi)

2. Oil for deep frying

3. Salt to suite your taste

4. Chili powder to suit your taste

5. Half teaspoon coriander powder

6. A pinch of cumin powder

Method

1. Take a big pot and boil the taro roots in fresh water. Keep boiling until the taro rots are soft.

2. Drain the water and cool the taro roots.

3. Peel them and slice them into about one millimeter to two millimeter thick slices.

4. Heat the oil, about two inches, in a thick-bottomed vessel. To test the oil, drop a slice of taro root into the oil. If the oil begins to bubble around it, the oil is ready to fry the chips.

5. Now drop the taro slices into the oil according to the size of the vessel. Do not overcrowd the vessel. Fry all the slices over medium flame, until the chips are crispy.

6. Stir the frying chips gently with a slotted ladle.

7. When the chips are of golden brown color, remove them from the oil and place them in a single layer on a paper towel to drain off the excess oil.

8. In this way, fry all the chips.

9. Sprinkle a little salt, cumin powder, chili powder, and coriander powder over the fried chips and serve them.

10.   Carrot Chips

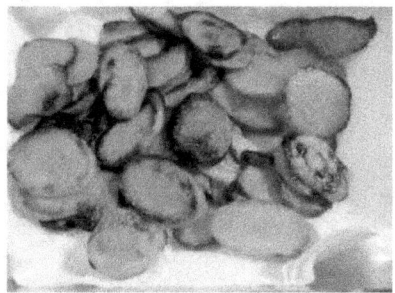

Required Ingredients

1. Four large peeled carrots, about an inch in diameter

2. Three teaspoons olive oil

3. One teaspoon kosher salt, or normal salt with a little large grains

4. Half a teaspoon black pepper powder

Method

1. Keep the oven preheated at about 180 degree Celsius. Arrange at least three of four racks in the oven if possible.

2. Cut the carrots in very thin slices, round. You can use a slicer to slice the chips.

3. Keep these carrot slices in a large bowl and sprinkle oil, salt, and pepper according to your taste.

4. Using your hands coat the carrots slices well with the oil and spices. See that the carrot slices are thoroughly coated.

5. Place the carrot slices in paper sheets in single layers. The chips can touch each other but they should not overlap each other. If there are more slices, you can bake them in a second batch.

23

6. Place the carrots slices in the preheated oven and bake them for about eight minutes. Switch off the oven.

7. Remove the chips from the trays and place them on the wire racks to cool until they are crisp. It will take about three to four minutes.

8. Remove the chips carefully with your hands and place them in a serving dish. You can use ranch dressing if you like.

9. You can store these chips in an air-tight container. They can be stored for about one week.

11. Spinach Chips

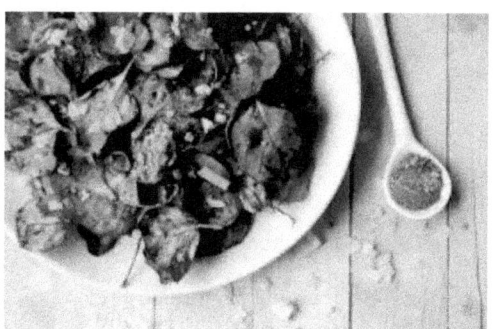

Required Ingredients

1. Four cups spinach, about 150 grams

2. One tablespoon olive oil

3. Salt to suit your taste

4. Black pepper to suit your taste

5. Italian herb seasoning (Optional)

Method

1. Keep the oven preheated at about 180 degree Celsius.

2. Put the spinach leaves in a large bowl and pour the oil over them. Now coat the leaves with oil using your hands.

3. Now add salt and the seasoning powder you like to suite your taste.

4. Mix everything properly. See that all the leaves get the salt and seasoning powder.

5. Spread a baking sheet and place the spinach leaves on the surface in single layer. They should not overlap.

6. Bake them for about ten to twelve minutes, until they are crispy.

7. Remove them from the oven and let them cool. Serve immediately.

12. Pear Chips

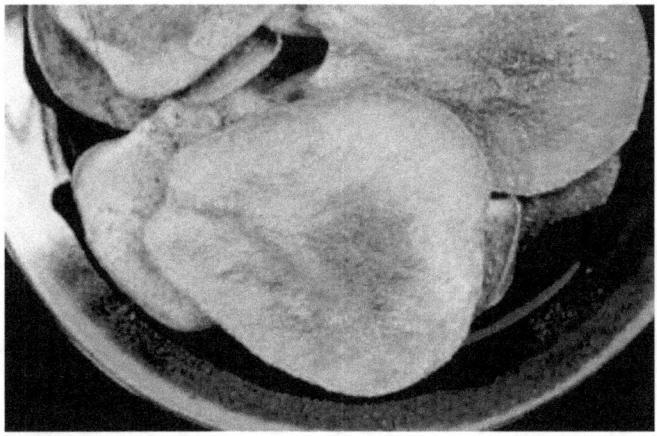

Required Ingredients

1. Four pears

2. Two tablespoons sugar

3. One teaspoon cinnamon powder

4. One-fourth teaspoon ground ginger

5. A pinch of red chili powder

Method

1. Preheat the oven to 150 degrees Celsius.

2. Wash and cut the pears into very thin slices. Remove the seeds and stems. Try to keep the slices as thin as possible. You can use a slicer if you like.

3. Spread the slices on a baking sheet in a single layer. You can use more than one baking sheet according to the racks you have in your oven.

4. The pears slices should not overlap.

5. Mix the sugar and the other spices in a small bowl. Adjust the spices according to your taste.

6. Sprinkle this spice mixture over the pears slices.

7. Bake these slices for about one hour. Turn them only once after about half an hour.

8. The chips will be ready when the edges of the chips will be a little curled.

9. Remove the chips from the oven and place them in a serving bowl or dish.

10. Serve the chips when they are completely cool. They will be crisp after cooling.

13. Apple Chips

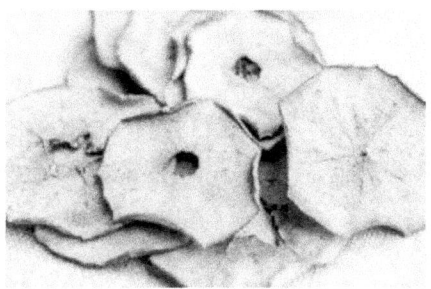

Required Ingredients

1. Two apples

2. Salt to suit your taste

3. Black pepper to suit your taste

Method

1. Wash and dry the apples.

2. Now cut the ends of the apples and make a deep hole in the middle and core out the middle part, including the seeds.

3. Now cut the apples into rounds as thin as possible. You can use a chips slicer to make very thin slices.

4. Place the sliced pieces on a baking paper. The pieces should not overlap.

5. If you have three or four wife racks in your oven, you can prepare three or four baking sheets. Otherwise, you will have to do it in batches.

6. Bake the chips at about 175 degrees Celsius for about five minutes.

7. When you see the edges beginning to curl up, flip each slice and bake them again for about one minute.

8. When the chips are crisp, remove them from the oven and put them in a serving dish.

9. Sprinkle salt and black pepper powder over the prepared chips. You can adjust salt and pepper according to your taste.

10. If you like you can use any seasoning herb that you like. Serve these chips immediately.

14. Cheese Chips

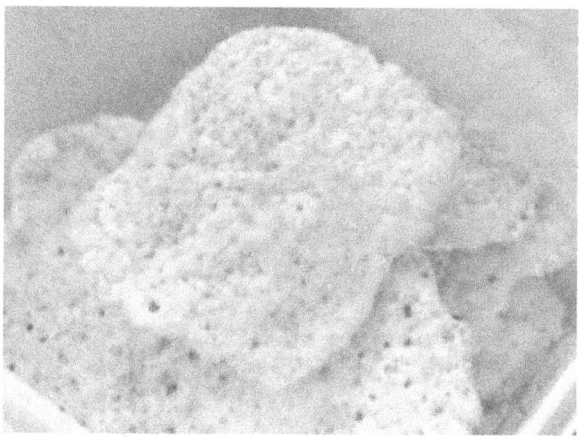

Required Ingredients

1. About 300 grams chunk of cheese

2. Salt and other spices to suite your taste

3. Herbs (optional)

Method

1. Keep an oven preheated at about 170 degrees Celsius.

2. Put a parchment paper over a baking sheet. Do not use waxed paper. Do not use silver foil.

3. Cut the cheese into very thin slices. Try to make about half millimeter thick slices. You can cut the cheese into small squares or strips.

4. You can also shred the cheese if you like.

5. Now place the square or long slices of the cheese on the parchment paper. See that they do not overlap. Leave some space between two slices because they will spread as they are baked.

6. Bake the slices for about six minutes.

7. When the edges of the slices begin to look brown, switch off the oven and let the chips remain inside the oven for about eight minutes.

8. They will become crispy. If you like you can sprinkle herbs, etc. but chesses is often salty so there is no need to add salt.

9. You can serve them when they are a little cool. You can enjoy these chips with your favorite dip.

15. Tofu Chips

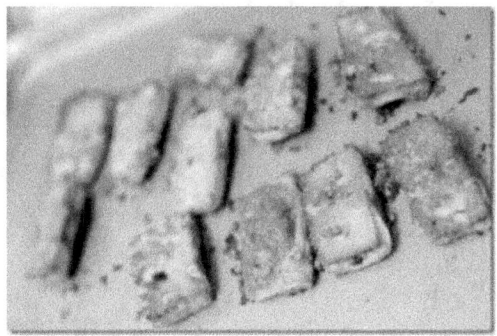

Required Ingredients

1. 400 grams very firm tofu

2. One fourth cup nutritional yeast

3. One fourth cup canola oil or any other oil you like to eat

Method

1. Cut the tofu into thin and small slices. You can make one inch squares. 2 mm thickness is enough.

2. Place these slices on a clean dishtowel and cover them with another dishtowel. The towels should be clean.

3. Now put a wooden board over the tofu slices and put some weight on top of the board to press the tofu slices. Leave the slices for about two hours.

4. After about two hours, apply nutritional yeast to the tofu slices. You can coat them with yeast from all sides.

5. Heat oil, about two inches, in a big skillet.

6. Now fry the tofu slices over low heat for about five minutes each side. Keep frying until the chips are crisp.

7. Remove the chips from the oil and place them on a paper towel to drain off the excess oil.

8. Serve them immediately.

16. Brinjal Chips

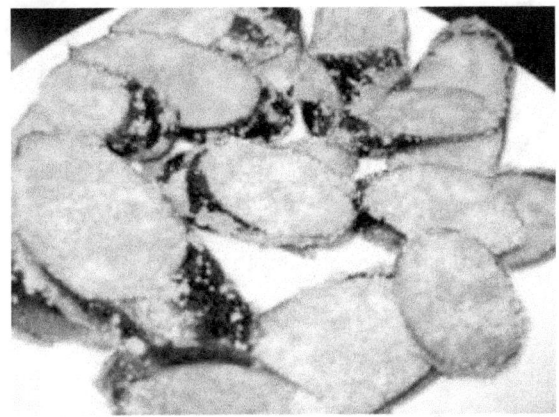

Required Ingredients

1. Six medium sized urinals (Eggplant)

2. Three teaspoons ginger garlic paste

3. Two teaspoons red chili powder, or according to your taste

4. Salt to suit your taste

5. A pinch of turmeric powder

6. One teaspoon oil for frying

Medium

1. Thinly slice the urinals in round shapes.

2. Put the urinals slices in a large bowl and add chili powder, turmeric powder, salt, and ginger garlic paste.

3. Coat the slices well with the spices and paste.

4. Apply very thin layer of paste on both sides of the slices.

31

5. Now heat the oil in a large frying pan and place the slices over the hot oil keeping a little distance from each other.

6. Now shallow fry the urinals slices from both sides. Keep turning them frequently.

7. Remove the fried slices from the oil and place them on paper towels for the excess oil to drain off.

8. Serve hot with tomato sauce or any other sauce you like.

17. Baked Turnip Chips

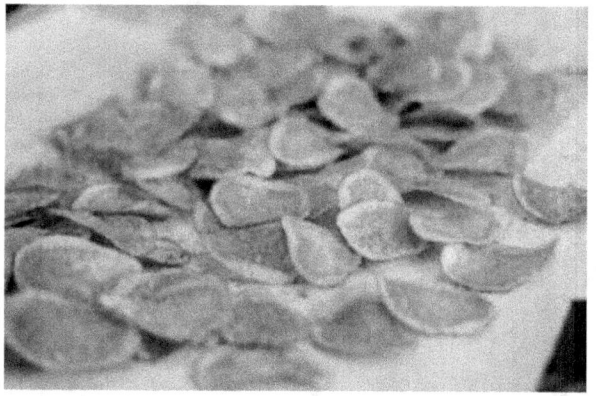

Required Ingredients

1. Three large peeled turnips

2. Four tablespoons olive oil, or any other oil you prefer

3. Half a teaspoon salt, or to suite your taste

4. One-fourth teaspoon pepper

Method

1. Keep an oven preheated at about 200 degrees Celsius.

2. Line the wire racks in the oven with two or three baking sheets with tin foils spread over them.

3. Gently spray the tin foils with cooking spray.

4. Using a sharp knife or a chips cutter, thinly slice the turnips into round chips. Do not cut them extremely thin.

5. Put the slices in a large bowl and add olive oil, salt, and pepper.

6. Toss them well so that they are coated with the oil and spices from all sides.

7. Now place the chips in a single layer on the baking sheets inside the oven. Do not overcrowd the sheets.

8. Bake the slices for about twenty five minutes. Turn them once after about 12 minutes.

9. Switch off the oven after about twenty five minutes, but do not remove the chips. Let them cool inside the oven for about 10 to 15 minutes so that they can become crisp.

10. Serve them immediately with any dip you like.

18. Beetroot Chips

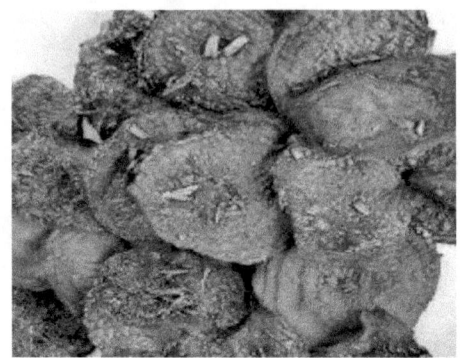

Required Ingredients

1. Two medium sized beetroots

2. One teaspoon olive oil

3. A little salt to suit your taste

4. Red chili powder to suite your taste

5. Black pepper to suit your taste

Method

1. Keep an oven preheated at about 180 degrees Celsius. It should have at least three racks.

2. Now peel the beetroots and slice them into about half mm thick rounds. You can use a chip slicer.

3. Put the slices in a large bowl and pour the olive oil over them. Add a little salt, red chili powder, and black pepper to suite your taste.

4. Toss the chips well so they are coated with oil and spices from all sides.

5. Now prepare two or three baking sheets. Place the beet slices in a single layer on the sheets. Keep the sheets into the oven and bake them for about twenty minutes.

6. When the edges of the beet slices are a little curled up, change the side of the chips and bake them again for about ten to twenty minutes.

7. When they are lightened in color, remove them from the oven and then place them on the wire rack. Switch off the oven after placing the chips on the wire racks. As they cool down, the chips will be crispy.

19. Kale Chips

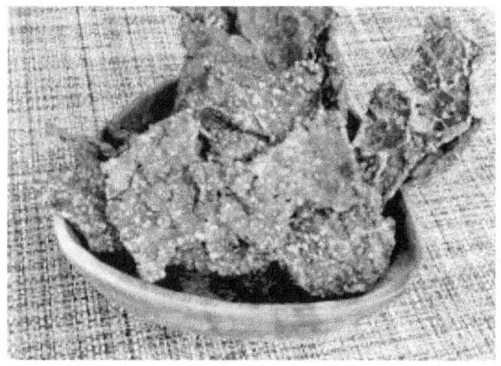

Required Ingredients

1. A bunch of raw kale cut into two or three inches pieces

2. One and a half tablespoons of olive oil

3. Half a teaspoon of kosher salt

4. One fourth teaspoon of black pepper powder

Method

1. Keep an oven preheated at about 165 degrees Celsius.

2. Put the kale pieces into a large bowl and pour the olive oil, salt, and pepper over the kale pieces.

3. Toss them well making it sure that the kale pieces are well-coated with oil and spices.

4. Now place the kale pieces on two or three baking sheets. Place them in a single layer.

5. See that the kale pieces do not overlap.

6. Bake the kale pieces for about twenty minutes. Check them once after about ten or twelve minutes.

7. When they are light brown and crispy, remove them from the oven and place them in a serving dish.

8. Serve them with tomato ketchup or any other dip you like.

20.French Fries

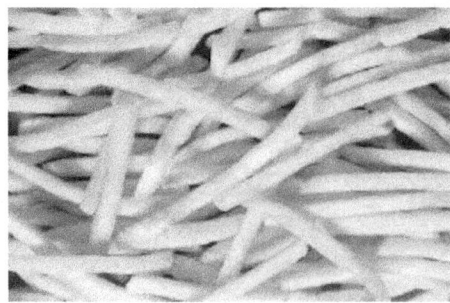

Required Ingredients

1. 500 grams potatoes

2. Oil for frying

3. Salt to suite your taste

4. A teaspoon Chat Masala or allspices

Method

1. Peel the potatoes with a potato peeler and keep them in water for some time.

2. Chop the peeled potatoes lengthways. You can use a French fry cutter if you do not want to cut the potatoes with a sharp knife.

3. Keep the potatoes pieces in water so that they do not become darker in color. Keep them in water for about five minutes. Excess starch will be removed from the potato pieces.

4. Now boil water in a deep pan and sink the potato pieces in the water when it begins to boil. Add a little salt to the water. You should boil the water only once.

5. Switch off the gas or store and let the potato pieces stay in the hot water for about five minutes.

6. Removed the potato pieces from the water and wipe them with a clean cotton cloth piece.

7. Put the potato pieces in your freezer for about 10 minutes.

8. Heat oil in a deep wok or a deep frying pan. There should be at least two inches of oil in the vessel.

9. When the oil is hot, put the potato pieces in the oil and remove them after frying them for just one minute.

10. Cool the fried potatoes for about two minutes. Keep the flame on so that the oil becomes hotter.

11. Now put the potato pieces back into the oil and keep frying them until they are a little brown.

12. Remove the French fries from the oil.

13. Place them in a serving dish. Sprinkle a little chat masala or allspices over them and mix them gently.

14. Serve these French fries with mayonnaise sauce, tomato sauce, or mint chutney.

21. Chunky Chips

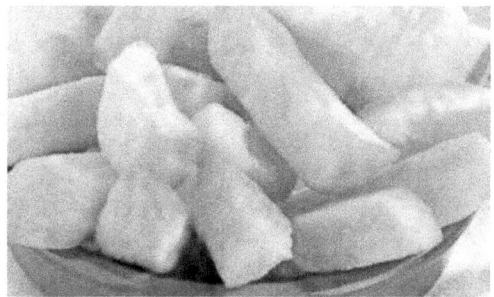

Required Ingredients

1. 1 kilo sweet potatoes

2. A little groundnut oil or any other oil you prefer

3. A little black salt and a little ground black pepper

Method

1. Keep an oven ready, preheated at about 235 degrees Celsius.

2. Peel the sweet potatoes and cut them into one centimeter wide slices. You can choose your own length of the potatoes.

3. Put the potato pieces in boiling water for about three minutes. Drain the water and remove the potato pieces.

4. Put the potatoes in a roasting pan and sprinkle a little oil over them. Toss them once or twice. See that the potatoes are well coated with the oil.

5. Now bake them in the preheated oven for about 20 minutes. Turn the potato pieces at least twice during the baking time.

6. Bake them until they are brown and crisp. Remove them from the oven and put them in a serving dish. Sprinkle a little salt and other herb if you like.

7. Serve the chunky chips with sauce of your preference.

22.Salt & Vinegar Banana Chips

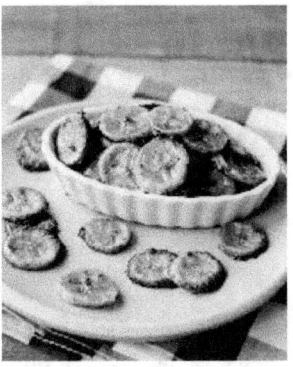

Ingredients for 2-3 servings

- Bananas

- 1 cup Malt Vinegar

- 2 tbsp. Olive Oil

- 1 tbsp. Sea Salt

Preparation – 30 to 40 minutes

1. Preheat the oven to 450 F (230 C).

2. Wash the bananas thoroughly and peel them.

3. Using the lowest (thinnest) setting on your mandolin slice the banana into rounds.

4. In a large bowl or a deep plate soak the freshly cut banana rounds in the malt vinegar and place in the refrigerator for at least 20 minutes.

5. After removing the soaking banana rounds from the refrigerator dry them off gently using paper towels.

6. Lightly drizzle 1 tbsp. Olive oil onto a baking tray.

7. Brush the remaining olive oil lightly onto both sides of the potato rounds and put on the baking tray.

8. Sprinkle a little sea salt on top of the banana rounds.

9. With the oven at temperature place the baking tray to bake for 15 to 20 minutes. Turn the chips over after 8 to 10 minutes. When the banana chips are golden and crisp they are ready to take out of the oven.

10. Remove the baking tray from the oven and with a plastic spatula remove the banana chips from the baking tray after allowing to cool for 2 minutes.

11. Serve and enjoy!

23. Thyme cucumber Chips

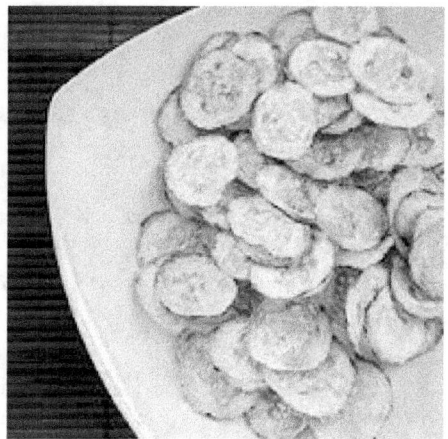

Ingredients for 4 servings

- 2 Large cucumbers

- 4 tbsp. Vegetable Oil

- 1 tsp. Dried Thyme

- 1 tsp. Sea Salt

Preparation – 30 to 40 minutes

1. Preheat the oven to 400 F (205 C).

2. Wash the cucumbers thoroughly.

3. Using the lowest (thinnest) setting on your mandolin slice the cucumbers into rounds and rinse in cold water afterwards

4. Lightly drizzle 2 tbsp. Vegetable oil onto a baking tray.

5. Place the cucumber rounds onto the baking tray and brush with 2 tbsp. of Vegetable oil. Take note not to stick the cucumber rounds on top of each other.

6. With the oven at temperature place the baking tray to bake for 15 to 20 minutes. Turn the chips over after 8 to 10 minutes. When the cucumber chips are golden and crisp they are ready to take out of the oven.

7. Remove the baking tray from the oven and sprinkle with the thyme and sea salt.

8. Remove the cucumber chips from the baking tray with a plastic spatula and serve after they have cooled for 5 minutes.

24. BBQ Zucchini Chips

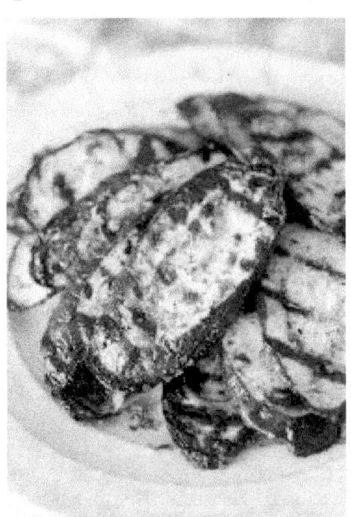

Ingredients for 2-3 servings

- Zucchini

- 4 cups cold water

- 1 tsp. Paprika

- 1/2 tsp. Garlic Salt

- 1/3 tsp. Sugar

- 1/3 tsp. Onion Powder

- Dash of Ground Mustard

- Dash of Cayenne Pepper

- Vegetable oil for frying

Method.

1. Wash zucchini.

2. Using the lowest (thinnest) setting on your mandolin slice the zucchini into rounds and rinse in cold water afterwards.

3. In a large bowl put the 4 cups of cold water and soak the zucchini rounds for half an hour.

4. In a small bowl or cup mix together the paprika, garlic salt, sugar, onion powder, ground mustard and cayenne pepper.

5. After removing the soaking zucchini rounds from the dry them off gently using paper towels.

6. Heat 1 to 2 inches (2.5 to 5 cm) of vegetable oil to 380 F (195 C) in an electric skillet or deep frying pan.

7. Fry the zucchini rounds for 2 minutes or until they are golden brown. Turn them over after the first minute.

8. Remove the zucchini chips from the electric skillet with a suitable slotted spoon and drain them on paper towels so there is no excess oil on them.

9. Sprinkle the mixture from the small bowl over the hot the zucchini chips.

10. Serve and enjoy!

25. Dill Onion Butternut Chips

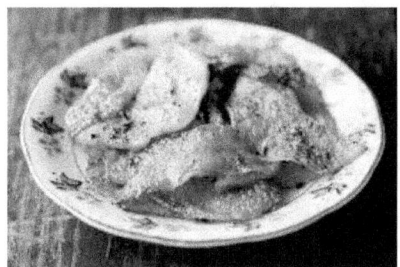

Ingredients for 4 servings

- 2 Large butternut

- 2 tbsp. Olive Oil

- 2 tsp. Onion powder

- 1 tsp. Dried Dill

- 1 tsp. Sea Salt

- 1 tbsp. Ground black pepper

Preparation – 30 to 35 minutes

1. Preheat the oven to 400 F (205 C).

2. Wash the butternuts thoroughly and peel them.

3. Using the lowest (thinnest) setting on your mandolin slice the butternuts into rounds and rinse in cold water afterwards.

4. Lightly drizzle 1 tbsp. olive oil onto a large baking tray.

5. Place the butternut rounds onto the baking tray and brush with 1 tbsp. of olive oil. Take note not to stick the butternut rounds on top of each other.

6. In a cup mix together the dill, onion powder, salt and pepper. Sprinkle this mixture over the butternut rounds on the baking tray.

7. With the oven at temperature place the baking tray to bake for 15 to 20 minutes. Turn the chips over after 8 to 10 minutes. When the butternut chips are golden and crisp they are ready to take out of the oven.

8. Remove the baking tray from the oven and leave to cool for 5 minutes.

9. Remove the butternut chips from the baking tray with a plastic spatula. If they are oily dry them with paper towels.

10. Serve and enjoy!

26. Red Thai Curry Coconut sweet Potato Chips

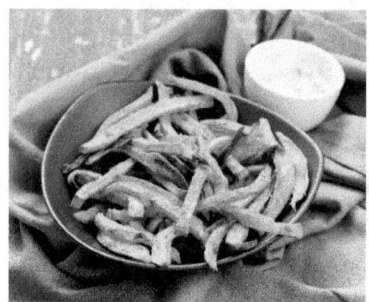

Ingredients for 4 servings

- 2 Large Sweet Potatoes (Ideally Red-Skinned, if not a Russet works fine)

- 4 tbsp. Vegetable Oil

- 1 tsp. Sea Salt

- 5 tbsp. Dried Coconut flakes

- Zest of 1 lime

- 2 tsp. Brown sugar

- 1 tsp. Freshly chopped lemon grass

- 1 tsp. Chili powder

- 1 tsp. Ginger powder

- 1/2 tsp. Garlic Powder

Preparation – 30 to 40 minutes Potato Chip Recipe

1. Preheat the oven to 400 F (205 C).

2. Wash the potatoes thoroughly. Do not peel them.

3. Using the lowest (thinnest) setting on your mandolin slice the potato into rounds and rinse in cold water afterwards. (Rinsing helps remove the starch, which aids with crisping during the bake). Drain and dry with paper towels afterwards.

4. Lightly drizzle 2 tbsp. Vegetable oil onto a baking tray.

5. Place the potato rounds onto the baking tray and brush with 2 tbsp. of Vegetable oil. Take note not to stick the potato rounds on top of each other.

6. With the oven at temperature place the baking tray to bake for 15 to 20 minutes. Turn the chips over after 8 to 10 minutes. When the potato chips are golden and crisp they are ready to take out of the oven.

7. Whilst the potato chips are still hot sprinkle the curry mixture over them.

Curry Powder Recipe

1. Place the dried coconut flakes, lime zest, brown sugar, freshly chopped lemongrass, ginger powder, garlic powder and chill powder into an electric blender. Blend thoroughly.

2. Sprinkle the curry powder onto the hot chips and serve.

27. *Wasabi Sweet Potato Chips*

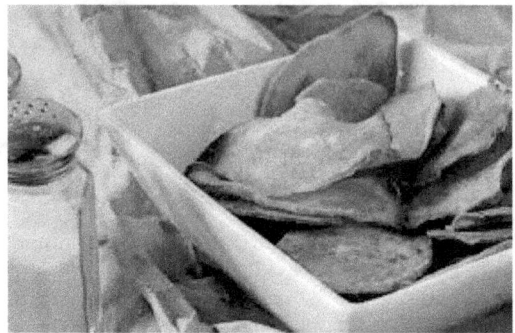

Ingredients for 4 servings

- 2 Sweet Potatoes (Ideally Red-Skinned, if not a Russet works fine)

- 2 tbsp. Olive Oil

- 2 tbsp. Wasabi Powder

- 1 1/2 tbsp. Sea Salt

- 2 tsp. Ground dried garlic

- 2 tsp. Sugar

- 1 tsp. Ground black pepper

- 1 tsp. Ground Ginger

Preparation – 45 to 50 minutes

1. Preheat the oven to 410 F (210 C).

2. Wash the potatoes thoroughly, no need to peel unless you prefer them without the skin.

3. Using the lowest (thinnest) setting on your mandolin slice the potatoes into rounds.

4. In a large bowl or a deep plate soak the freshly cut potato rounds in cold water for 10 minutes to remove the starch.

5. After removing the soaking potato rounds dry them off gently using paper towels.

6. Lightly drizzle 2 tbsp. Olive oil onto a baking tray.

7. In a large bowl mix together 1/2 tsp. of ground ginger, 1 tbsp. of Wasabi powder, 1 tsp. of ground garlic, 1 tsp. of sugar and 1 tbsp. of salt. Add the potato rounds and mix together.

8. Put the potato rounds onto the baking tray and put into the now hot oven for 20 to 25 minutes. Do not stack the rounds on top of each other.

9. Turn the chips over after 10 to 12 minutes. When the potato chips are golden and crisp they are ready to take out of the oven.

10. Remove the baking tray from the oven and with a plastic spatula remove the potato chips from the baking tray after allowing to cool for 2 minutes.

11. Mix the remaining spices in a small bowl or cup and sprinkle over the potato chips.

12. Serve and enjoy!

28. Easy Pita Bread Chips

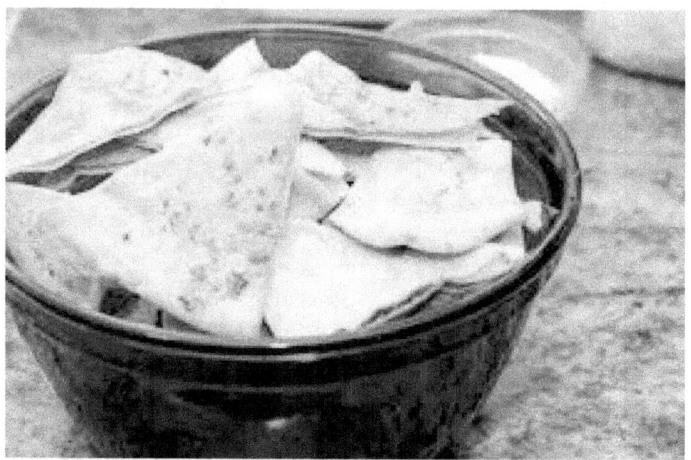

Here is an easy cheat's pita bread chip recipe. This is a great way to use up old pita breads before they go out of date.

Ingredients for 4 servings

- 10 Pita Bread pockets

- 1/2 cup Virgin Olive Oil

- 1 tsp. Ground Garlic

- 1 tsp. Freshly chopped Parsley

- 1/2 tsp. Dried Basil

- 1/2 tsp. Ground black pepper

Preparation – 20 minutes

1. Preheat the oven to 410 F (210 C).

2. With a sharp knife cut the pita bread pockets into 8 triangles.

3. Lightly drizzle 1 tbsp. Virgin Olive oil onto a baking tray and place the pita triangles onto the baking tray.

4. In a bowl mix together the virgin olive oil, the parsley, the basil, the sea salt and the garlic.

5. Brush the mixture over all of the pita bread triangles.

6. Put the baking tray in the oven and bake for 8 to 10 minutes, turning the pita bread triangles over after 4 to 5 minutes.

7. When the pita chips should be brown and crispy remove them from the oven.

8. Allow to cool for 2 minutes. Serve.

29. Spicy Sweet Potato Chips

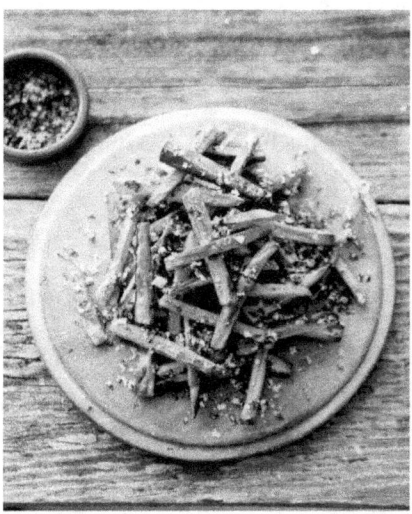

A spicy twist on the traditional sweet potato chip will please the men in the house.

Ingredients for 4 servings

- 3 Large Sweet Potatoes

- 2 tbsp. Olive Oil

- 2 tbsp. Maple Syrup

- 1 tsp. Sea Salt

- 1/2 tsp. Cayenne Pepper

Preparation – 30 to 35 minutes

1. Preheat the oven to 450 F (230 C).

2. Wash the sweet potatoes thoroughly. Do not peel them.

3. Using the lowest (thinnest) setting on your mandolin slice the sweet potato into thin rounds.

4. In a small bowl or cup mix together the maple syrup, olive oil and cayenne pepper.

5. Drizzle a little olive oil onto a baking tray.

6. Brush the maple syrup mixture onto both sides of the sweet potato rounds and place them on the baking tray.

7. Lightly sprinkle the salt and pepper on the sweet potato rounds.

8. Sprinkle a little sea salt on top of the potato rounds.

9. With the oven at temperature place the baking tray to bake for 15 to 20 minutes. Turn the chips over after 8 to 10 minutes. When the sweet potato chips are golden and crisp they are ready to take out of the oven.

10. Remove the baking tray from the oven and with a plastic spatula remove the potato chips from the baking tray after allowing to cool for 2 minutes.

11. Serve and enjoy!

30. Smokey Parmesan Sweet Potato Chips

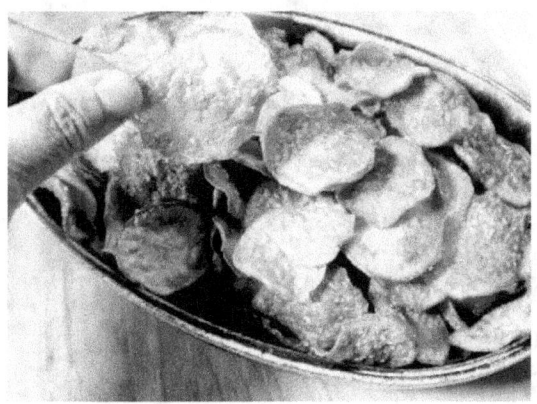

These Smokey Parmesan sweet potato chips will leave you wanting more.

Ingredients for 4 servings

- 1 Large Sweet Potato (Or 2 medium)

- 1/2 cup Freshly grated Parmesan Cheese

- 2 tbsp. Olive Oil

- 2 tsp. Sea Salt

- 1 tsp. Smoked Paprika

- 1 tsp. Ground Black Pepper

- 1/2 tsp. Garlic powder

Preparation – 30 to 35 minutes

1. Preheat the oven to 380 F (195 C).

2. Wash and peel the sweet potato.

3. Using the lowest (thinnest) setting on your mandolin slice the sweet potato into thin rounds.

4. In a small bowl or cup mix together the freshly grated Parmesan cheese, the sea salt, smoked paprika, black pepper and garlic powder. Syrup.

5. In a large bowl mix the potato rounds with the olive oil.

6. When well mixed add the Parmesan cheese mixture and mix once more.

7. Drizzle a little olive oil onto a baking tray and place a single layer of the potato rounds.

8. When the oven is at temperature place the baking tray in and bake for 20 to 25 minutes. Turn the chips over after 10 to 12 minutes.

9. Remove the baking tray from the oven and with a plastic spatula remove the potato chips from the baking tray after allowing to cool for 2 minutes.

10. Serve and enjoy!

31. Baked Orange & Thyme Sweet Potato Chips

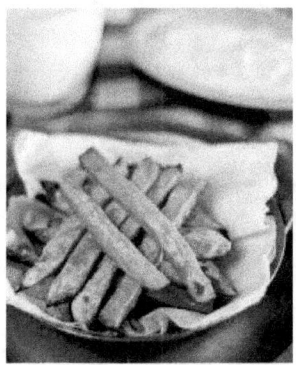

These zesty delights will impress all of your friends and family.

Ingredients for 4 servings

- 2 Large Sweet Potatoes

- 5 tbsp. Virgin Olive Oil

- 1/2 cup Freshly squeezed Orange juice

- 1 tbsp. Orange Zest

- 1 tbsp. Thyme

- 1 tsp. Sea Salt

Preparation – 35 to 35 minutes

1. Preheat the oven to 320 F (160 C).

2. Wash the sweet potatoes but do not peel them.

3. Using the lowest (thinnest) setting on your mandolin slice the sweet potatoes into thin rounds.

4. In a bowl mix together the virgin olive oil, the orange juice, the orange zest and the thyme.

5. Drizzle some virgin olive oil on a baking tray.

6. Dip or brush the sweet potato rounds with the oil mixture and put the potato rounds onto the baking tray. Do not stack the rounds on top of each other.

7. Sprinkle the sweet potato rounds with the sea salt and put the baking tray in the oven for 20 to 25 minutes. Turn the rounds over after 10 to 12 minutes.

8. When the chips are brown and crispy from the baking tray from the oven.

9. Let the chips cool for 4 to 5 minutes before serving.

32. Fried Cinnamon Sweet Potato Chips

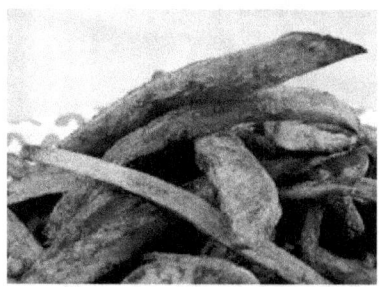

One of the few fried chip recipes in this book, these are worth the effort.

Ingredients for 4 servings

- 2 Large Sweet Potatoes

- 1/2 cup All Purpose Flour

- 1/2 cup Milk

- 1 1/2 tbsp. Sugar (Refined white sugar is preferred)

- 1 tsp. Ground Ginger

- 1 1/2 tsp. Ground Cinnamon

- 1 1/2 tsp. Sea Salt

- Vegetable oil for frying

Preparation – 20 to 55 minutes

1. Wash the sweet potatoes thoroughly.

2. Using the lowest (thinnest) setting on your mandolin slice the sweet potato into thin rounds.

3. Place the sweet potato rounds into a large bowl and add the milk so that the rounds soak up the milk.

4. In a small bowl mix together the flour, ground ginger, 1 tsp. ground cinnamon, 1 tbsp. sugar and 1 tsp. Sea salt.

5. Dip the sweet potato rounds into the cinnamon mix and then place them on a plate.

6. Heat 1 to 2 inches (2.5 to 5 cm) of vegetable oil to 380 F (195 C) in an electric skillet or deep frying pan.

7. Fry the sweet potato rounds for 2 minutes or until they are golden brown. Turn them over after the first minute.

8. Remove the potato chips from the electric skillet with a suitable slotted spoon and drain them on paper towels so there is no excess oil on them.

9. In a small bowl or cup mix together 1/2 tbsp. sugar, 1/2 tsp. sea salt and 1/2 tsp. of cinnamon.

10. Sprinkle the sugar cinnamon mixture on the hot sweet potato chips.

11. Serve and enjoy!

33. Chipotle Sweet Potato Chips

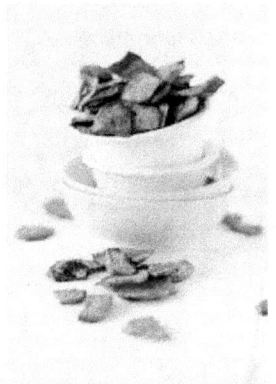

(Microwave Recipe) These tasty sweet potato chips are cooked in the microwave. Take care to verify the power of your microwave so that you can adjust the timings if necessary.

Ingredients for 4 servings

- 3 Medium size Sweet Potatoes

- 2 tbsp. Olive Oil

- 1 1/2 tbsp. Garlic Powder

- 1 tbsp. Sea Salt

- 2 tsp. Smoked Paprika

- 1/2 tsp. Chili powder

- 1/2 tsp. Chipotle Chili Powder

Preparation – 10 to 20 minutes

1. Wash the sweet potatoes thoroughly.

2. Using the lowest (thinnest) setting on your mandolin slice the sweet potato into thin rounds.

3. Put the sweet potato rounds in a large bowl and toss with the sea salt and olive oil.

4. On a plate suitable for use in your microwave put parchment paper and place the sweet potato rounds on the plate. Don't allow the rounds to overlap. Note, you will either need to prepare a couple of plates or reuse the plate several times to cook all of the chips.

5. Microwave the sweet potato rounds on high for 4 to 5 minutes (based on a 1000W microwave, adjust time accordingly).

6. In a small bowl mix together the garlic powder, chipotle chili powder, paprika and chill powder.

7. When the sweet potato chips have finished cooking in the microwave (they should be crisp, if not microwave for an additional minute or two) remove from the microwave and sprinkle with the chipotle mixture.

8. Repeat steps 4 to 7 until all of the chips have cooked.

9. Allow the chips to cool for 2 to 3 minutes, then serve!

34. Baked Carrot Chips

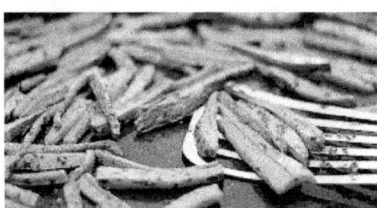

Baked carrot chips provide a healthy and tasty alternative to potato chips. This are so simple to prepare your children could easily do them for you.

Ingredients for 2 servings

- 2 Large Carrots

- 2 tbsp. Virgin Olive Oil

- 1/2 tsp. Sea Salt

Preparation – 20 to 25 minutes

1. Preheat the oven to 360 F (180 C).

2. Wash the carrots thoroughly and then peel them.

3. Using the lowest (thinnest) setting on your mandolin slice the carrots into rounds.

4. Drizzle 1 tbsp. of virgin olive oil on a baking tray.

5. Place the carrot rounds on the baking tray and drizzle the remaining 1 tbsp. of virgin olive oil on top and lightly season with the sea salt.

6. When the oven is at temperature place the baking tray in the oven and bake for 15 to 20 minutes. Turn the chips over after 8 to 10 minutes.

7. When the edges of the carrot appear to be crispy they are ready to be removed from the oven.

8. Let the carrot chips cool for a couple of minutes and then serve.

35. Spicy Carrot Chips

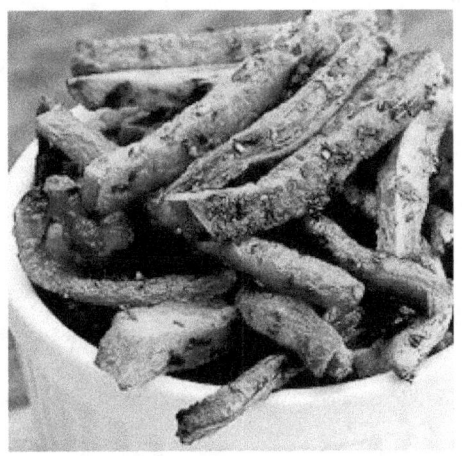

These make a real healthy treat with a kick.

Ingredients for 4 servings

- 4 Large Carrots

- 1 tbsp. Olive Oil

- 1 tbsp. Coconut Oil

- 1 tsp. Ground Black Pepper

- 1 tsp. Cayenne Pepper

- 1/2 tsp. Sea Salt

Preparation – 20 to 25 minutes

1. Preheat the oven to 380 F (195 C).

2. Wash the Carrots and then peel them.

3. Using the lowest (thinnest) setting on your mandolin slice the carrots into rounds.

4. Drizzle the olive oil on a baking tray.

5. In a small bowl mix together the coconut oil with the ground pepper, cayenne pepper and sea salt.

6. Dip the carrot rounds in the spice mixture and then place them on the baking tray. Note, only one layer of carrots, do not stack them.

7. When the oven is at temperature place the baking tray in the oven and bake for 15 to 20 minutes. Turn the chips over after 8 to 10 minutes.

8. When the edges of the carrots appear to be crispy they are ready to be removed from the oven.

9. Let the spicy carrot chips cool for a couple of minutes and then serve.

36.Baked Eggplant Chips

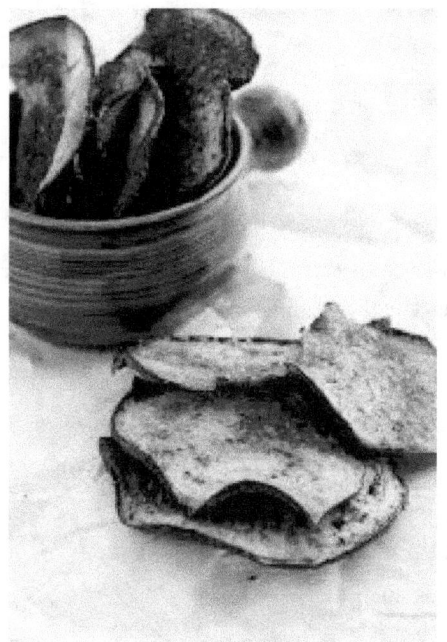

Simply delicious!

Ingredients for 4 servings

- 1 Large Eggplant

- 1/2 cup bread crumbs

- 1/4 cup Grated Parmesan cheese

- 2 tbsp. Olive Oil

- 1 tbsp. Freshly chopped or ground garlic

- 2 Freshly chopped Parsley sprigs

- 1 tsp. Dried Oregano

- 1/2 tsp. Sea Salt

Preparation – 40 to 45 minutes

1. Preheat the oven to 220 F (105 C).

2. Wash the eggplant thoroughly. Do not peel them.

3. Using the lowest (thinnest) setting on your mandolin slice the eggplants lengthwise into strips.

4. Drizzle 1 tbsp. of olive oil on a baking tray.

5. Place the eggplant strips on the baking tray and drizzle the remaining 1 tbsp. of olive oil on top and lightly season with the sea salt.

6. In a small bowl mix together the Parmesan cheese, the bread crumbs, the parsley, the oregano, the garlic and the salt. Sprinkle this mixture over the eggplant strips.

7. When the oven is at temperature place the baking tray in the oven and bake for 25 to 30 minutes. Turn the eggplant strips over after 12 to 15 minutes.

8. When the edges of the eggplant appear to be crispy they are ready to be removed from the oven.

9. Let the eggplant chips cool for a couple of minutes and then serve.

Conclusion

In a nutshell, the Keto Diet is a low-carbohydrate, high fat and modest protein nutritional plan that uses the process of ketosis to accelerate the rate at which fats are burned by the body.

Science behind the diet

Typically, when the body requires energy, it will burn sources of carbohydrates first which are turned into glucose and processed throughout the body. This process is particularly helpful with brain function and can be evidenced by the fact that, without a source of quality carbohydrates, we can feel a little sluggish in our mind. With the Ketogenic Diet being low in the principle energy source, the body has to find alternative supplies; this is where the diet part kicks in. Without carbohydrates, the liver looks instead to fat and turns these into fatty acids and Ketone bodies. The brain can use these Ketones as a replacement for glucose and continue to function while the body goes into a state of ketosis. It is in this state that fat is burned at a higher rate.

FREE Bonus Reminder

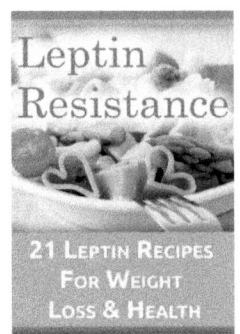

If you have not grabbed it yet, please go ahead and download your special bonus report *"Leptin Resistance. 21 Leptin Recipes For Weight Loss & Healthy Living"*.

Simply Click the Button Below

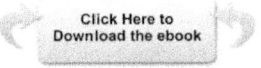

OR **Go to This Page**

http://easyweightlossway.com/free/

BONUS #2: More Free Books

Do you want to receive more Free Books?

We have a mailing list where we send out our new Books when they go free on Kindle. Click on the link below to sign up for Free Book Promotions. => Sign Up for Free Book Promotions <=

OR Go to this URL http://bit.ly/1V4Xan7

www.ingramcontent.com/pod-product-compliance
Lightning Source LLC
Chambersburg PA
CBHW071115280526
45787CB00003B/1056